Thyroid Conditions and Interesting Medical Subjects

By: James M. Lowrance © 2018

I0505465

TABLE OF CONTENTS:

ONE

How Important it is to Test for Thyroid Antibodies

Recently my wife had a visit with a doctor who tested her for thyroid hormone imbalance. I told her before she even went, that the doctor would test her "TSH" only, which stands for "Thyroid Stimulating Hormone". This is the hormone sent from the pituitary gland that regulates the amount of the hormone that is sent to the thyroid gland, for getting it to produce the proper amount of its own hormones. Everyone's thyroid gland changes throughout the day regarding how much stimulation by the pituitary is needed. Certain foods, a change in physical activity and other factors can cause the thyroid gland to increase or decrease the sending-out of its own hormones throughout the body.

The hormones from the thyroid gland, consisting mainly of "T-4" (Thyroxine") and T-3 ("Triiodothyronine") are what regulate the body's metabolism in all organs and even in all cells of the body. These fluctuations cause the pituitary to either back off a bit or increase a bit in the amount of TSH it sends to the thyroid, within the normal range set by the testing lab. While this is certainly well and fine to test the TSH level (very sensitive and accurate), by only testing it this likely misses millions of cases of developing thyroid disease. Possibly therefore the National Institutes of Health states that about half of thyroid disease cases remain undiagnosed.

The T-3 and T-4 should be tested (a "Thyroid Panel") as well but something of little known importance that should also be tested as well, are "Thyroid Antibodies", mainly being the "Anti-TPO" (anti Thyroid peroxidase) and the "Anti-TG" ("Anti Thyroglobulin").

Why are these tests important? Because they can become elevated before thyroid hormones become imbalanced, resulting in a condition of hyperthyroidism called Grave's disease or in a condition of hypothyroidism called Hashimoto's thyroiditis.

Grave's will manifest even in developing/initial stages with the thyroid hormones being in lower range or borderline low but with clinically elevated thyroid antibodies. These antibodies should not be present at all except in very low incidental titers (lab detection measurements). When Grave's becomes clearly detectable in the hormones and TSH (clinically low titers), a patient will be diagnosed with Grave's disease, which speeds up everything in a person's metabolism. First-line treatment is often "anti-thyroid drugs", which help to lower elevated thyroid hormones.

With high-normal or borderline-high tested TSH and even slightly-low thyroid hormone levels, plus a showing of these same thyroid antibodies, the opposite condition of a slowed-down metabolism will begin to occur, called "hypothyroidism", which results in all bodily cells becoming sluggish and requiring treatment. The treatment is opposite from that of a sped-up metabolism that is caused by Grave's disease and in the case of hypothyroidism; most cases caused by Hashimoto's thyroiditis, the treating physician will prescribe thyroid hormones that raise below-normal readings of them, back into the normal range. The pituitary gland is no longer able to do so on its own because the thyroid gland has become diseased.

So, why test for thyroid antibodies? The answer is obvious; because thyroid disease can be brewing inside a person's body but the thyroid hormones themselves are not yet reflecting this!

I have written to a fair extent about how thyroid disease can affect nerve and muscle function. In one of the smaller books I took 6 detailed Q&A and made the booklet from them. "Thyroid Neuropathy and Myopathy Questions and Answers" is the title of that resource. I took the 6 questions from among those I have received through correspondence from thyroid patients, over the past decade or so (Since about 2004). I then compiled them into the booklet with relatively detailed answers. The questions that were asked of me were mostly those I received by email, from members of fellow patient support forums and message boards where I was moderator. They obtained my private email address of that time, by request. While I am not a medical professional, these fellow patients knew I was well-studied as a layperson but that most importantly "I had been there". I had been and was in some of the same situations they were corresponding with me about. When some of these forums were discontinued and taken offline (not by hosting companies but by the owners of the websites), I gleaned some of my better forum responses on the thyroid-related myopathy and neuropathy subjects from them as well as from email correspondence previously-described.

These are represented under the 'Q and A' headings within the booklet. Among the subjects of discussion that took place between me and these other thyroid patients, were symptoms of thyroid myopathy and/or neuropathy (the former being muscle weakness and the latter being nerve damage causing a variety of symptoms including pain). I am well-informed about the types of testing that were administered to me personally when I was being diagnosed with both myopathy and peripheral neuropathy. I have gained knowledge regarding these thyroid-related issues and the prognoses that can usually be expected from treatments for them (how patients respond to the treatments). Within the discussions, I talk about blood tests and sometimes overlooked deficiencies of nutrients that can cause neuropathies and myopathies, which thyroid disease patients (and diabetics) are more susceptible to. I also look at both hypothyroid (underactive) and hyperthyroid (overactive) conditions, both of which can contribute to these symptom-problems of muscle weakness and nerve pain. Special types of testing involved in diagnosing these problems are also a point of discussion, including the QSART test, EMG and nerve/muscle biopsy testing. These discussions are for fellow-patient support and general educational purposes and that thyroid patients should always follow their doctor's orders. Being armed with some degree of knowledge in these areas, however, can help patients better discuss with their doctors, their options for controlling symptoms. Some patients may even overcome these manifestations of muscle weakness and nerve pain completely over time. This depends on correctable comorbid illnesses; additional hormone imbalances and/or vitamin deficiencies being treated. In some cases, physical therapy can restore muscle function considerably in some patients.

TWO

Can Heart Skips be Dangerous to Your Cardiac Health?

This answer I gave to a man who was experiencing forceful heart-skip palpations, I believe holds answers for others who have this same <u>usually benign</u> heart symptom. A link to one of my books on this subject is in red-bold, at the end of this article. - - -

I'm truly sorry you're having to put up with those crazy PVCs and the breath-drop which I have too! They are disturbing to say the least. I've been to two cardiologists (I strongly recommend you go to at least one) and I told them my PVCs come forcefully at times and cause me to cough or breath slightly differently for a few seconds. They both told me that these heart skip palpitations can be related to heart problems but very rarely. In these rare cases they are not a cause either but a symptom (such as mild leakage from the Mitral Valve). They also said that large numbers of people come to them with these and their hearts check out completely normal. They may, however, be diagnosed with common Mitral Valve Prolapse that's symptomatic (syndrome).

This has caused many doctors to believe they are mostly stress and anxiety related, even if you feel them forcefully or don't feel them at all (Many people have them and don't even know it!). They also said that flutters are often related to these but that unless a person has a sustained flutter or even episodes in which a flutter occurs for quite a few seconds, that this too is not immediately harmful but still worthy of having checked -

especially if sustained episodes are experienced. They call this Atrial Fibrillation (A-Fib) that's treated with medications and lifestyle modifications (e.g. improved diet and regular exercise to tolerance level and medication). Even with the later mentioned, medications literally allow a sufferer to carry on their lives as if they don't have the condition and their life-expectancy is basically that of people without A-Fib.

In short, I leaned that the heart skips alone; which are premature skips that combine with a regular heartbeat, are in the vast majority of cases, of no significant value in heart disease diagnoses. Some even reputable sites (far outnumbered by those that state otherwise), say that PVCs place a person at risk for sudden cardiac arrest. However, if this were true, because a large percent of the population has them, whether they feel them or not, people would be dropping dead left and right, young and old, every day in the world. This simply is not happening as a cause of death - it is not of itself a heart disease, apart from A-Fib which is unmistakable when experienced and highly regulate-able.

THREE

Septoplasty I Underwent to Correct Deviated Septum and Nasal Breathing

Because of my having moderate non-smoker's CODP (more common than most people think), my pulmonologist told me that I should have my sinuses checked out by an ENT doctor (Nose, Ears and Throat Specialist), to make sure I didn't have something like sinus drainage at night, which can build in your lungs and cause a worse morning cough. Just to make a definition clarification – "adult onset asthma" is when you have some lung obstruction that is at least to some degree "reversible". That just means that when they administer a Bronchodilator during PFTs (pulmonary function tests), it will open some of the obstructed breathing. During my tests, mine only improved by about 1% after Bronchodilator and the percent of reversed obstruction, needs to be about 12% to diagnose lung obstruction as "asthma" (with strong confidence). This is not an absolute however, and different spirometer normal values (breathing test machines), use different sets of numbers, due to a patient's weight/BMI, etc... What the ENT doctor found regarding me, via a head-only CT scan, was that I had a "deviated septum", requiring an operation to correct it for better breathing through my nose (septoplasty).

The "deviation' seen on the tests means it was pushed too far to one side and needed straightened back out. When the middle of this cartilage in the nose is pushed to one side, which can be the case at birth or from injury at some point, it not only makes kind of a bulge toward one nostril, cutting off partial or all breathing on that side but if the deviation is in the middle of it, it can make an

"S"-shape, partially cutting off breathing to both nostrils. Mine was pushing mostly to the right side, so much so, that on CT x-ray, it looked like an arrow or a vertical "V" pressing my right nostril outwardly a bit and not allowing much air to come into it. This caused me dry mouth with exercise and when sleeping at night. Proper nose-breathing is important because it better exchanges the oxygen and carbon dioxide in the lungs. It's possible that mine occurred or was worsened if present at birth, when I was injured about 13 years ago (in year 2001), when my son and I were topping trees at a mobile home park we managed in West Oklahoma for 2.5 years.

We were unloading a full-size U-Haul truck full of large limbs, when like an idiot, I pulled on one to dislodge it and it hit me smack in the nose! The impact was such that Zac and I found by glasses about 20 feet behind me. I held my nose and told him "don't look.... don't look!" because I could feel sticks protruding from my nose and thought it was broken bone or cartridge. His main concern was to keep asking me "It's not your eye is it dad?!" I kept telling him it was only my nose but when I got home, I had to dig 3 pieces of stick out of the flesh of my left nostril. Also, like an idiot, I didn't go to the doctor at that time and it left me with a notch on the rim of my nostril, that needed sewed up (you can barely see it today) but the main damage was inside my nose. I feel this may have...actually very likely did contribute to my nose cartilage problem – my deviated septum.

My operation went well but left me with a little more pain than I expected and lots of bleeding, with need to change bandages a lot (I know gross!). That's why I didn't take a pic of it because it was also stitched-up and I had two splint type devices – one inside each nostril that was taken after one week. I didn't even show my wife Jan, the nose when not bandaged because it was slightly pugged, so I looked different. I told her I look like James Cagney when he plays a gangster in the old movies "Mmmm, you're the guy that got my brother, now I'm the guy who's going to get you - mmmm". So, that's my nose job story, which was performed on me 08/18/2014. I have since recovered from the operation with moderate satisfaction in nose-breathing.

FOUR

Stop Catastrophic Anxiety Disorder Thoughts with Humor

In my eBook on Amazon titled "Chronic Anxiety Unreality Symptoms", I touch about taking catastrophic thoughts and converting them into humor. These thoughts are what some people refer to as "what if thinking" which can consist of terrible and disturbing thoughts and fear of catastrophic events taking place. Many anxiety sufferers experience this type of thinking and many times their thoughts come from the fear of losing control and committing violent acts. These thoughts are irrational and the fact that they are disturbing to the person experiencing them, means they will not act upon them. They are simply phobias with no true basis, but they can of course still be greatly concerning. This is especially true when they serve to trigger panic attacks or what we also call the "fight or flight response". So, how do you add humor to these types of thoughts or convert them into funny scenarios that take the threat out of them? Well, it's certainly not always easy to do but something anxiety sufferers can work on that may yield them good success in diverting these phobic thoughts away from their original irrational direction.

Some anxiety sufferers may simply replace these thoughts with different ones which can also be effective, and they may not always use humor to do so (Whatever works!). I did want to give further description however of how humor can replace catastrophic thinking because this question was specifically asked by a reader of one of the chapters of my books on the catastrophic thinking subject. I add more suggestion in the following paragraphs but also want to remind that "what if" thoughts are common with anxiety disorders and they do not indicate that the one experiencing them is going to snap or lose touch with reality. You could say they are phantom thoughts that have no true basis and will not actually cause us harm. What a great question it was that a reader recently asked and one I really appreciate them asking and that was his wanting to know specifically how to implement diversionary thinking into thoughts about snapping and becoming violent to others. A few years ago, I ordered a man's eBook online that printed-out on my copy machine (his method for delivering it). I don't remember the book or author's name but gave it to my son who also suffers anxiety.

I do remember the author talking about having the bizarre thought that he would suddenly pick up a knife and start stabbing people around him. He described the thought in such a way that made me laugh and I found appreciation in that. I don't remember exactly what type humor he injected into this paragraph, but it worked and made me realize that this was a great method for thought-diversion in turning catastrophic thoughts into something to laugh at, thereby rendering it powerless to increase anxiety states. Some ideas I would suggest is to change the thought of a knife in your hand into a fish and how funny it would be to attack someone with a limp fish. If the thought that you'll point a gun at someone enters your mind, picture shooting bubbles out of it rather than bullets. While someone without anxiety might see these as ridiculous suggestions, they are legitimate methods in my opinion for turning the tables on anxiety and beating it at its own game.

It may sound like I'm placing anxiety into a category of being an enemy we have to defeat but we are simply working on mastering it, so that it works for us instead of against us. We do see anxiety as an enemy when it is "busting us" so-to-speak and causing us aguish. Our goal is rather to see anxiety provide us more energy and inspiration to accomplish things in our lives and that is when we become a partner to its true purpose and can then call anxiety a friend instead of a foe.

FIVE

My Books on Adrenal Fatigue

In these books I include vital details regarding Adrenal Fatigue symptoms, diagnosis and treatments. Written by me, a fellow sufferer who experiences this stress syndrome after prolonged periods of stress (chronic) or from sudden, severe stress episodes (traumatic). I, the author has also found treatments and lifestyle change methods that have been tremendously effective in relieving my symptoms. In year-2003, I began developing autoimmune thyroid disease (Hashimoto's Thyroiditis), plus I was going through a prolonged, severe period of stress. I began to experience this very real syndrome which results in diminished adrenal function at a subclinical level - not full blown hypoadrenalism (Addison's disease), which is very severe and that can be life threatening as well. I was attended by doctors who diagnosed my subclinical adrenal dysfunction, through testing which revealed that the low functioning adrenal syndrome was co-morbid (co-occurring) to my Hashimoto's thyroid disease. Since Adrenal Fatigue is a sub-clinical condition and not full-blown adrenal failure, many doctors will not recognize it as a legitimate illness and therefore not treat the syndrome. However highly reputable medical research studies have been published that describe subclinical adrenal dysfunction that is associated with certain illnesses and stress syndromes. Some of the diseases and syndromes that may result in Adrenal Fatigue, or that may include it as a comorbid feature of them, include Chronic Fatigue Syndrome (CFS), Fibromyalgia (FMS), Post-Traumatic Stress Disorder (PTSD) and autoimmune and inflammatory diseases of all types. Most people suffering from

Adrenal Fatigue began experiencing the adrenal dysfunction due to chronic stress rather than it being due to other co-morbid health conditions. Some sufferers refer to the symptoms of mild adrenal hypo functioning as feeling like they are "stressed out" most of the time.

There is hope for recovery and some patients will see full recovery and future prevention of the illness from re-occurring. The importance, however, is becoming well-educated about this often-debilitating health disorder, this will help sufferers see the best results from treatment and the recovery of a better life quality. These books contain realistic warnings regarding cortisol treatments for Adrenal Fatigue (cortical steroids) but they ARE NOT "anti-cortisol" regarding the possible options for treatment. What I state is the fact that non-steroidal treatment is preferred and should be attempted first, due to the potentially serious side-effects corticosteroids can cause in people who do not have Addison's disease, which is full blown adrenal dysfunction. I also state in these books that if cortical dosing is administered, there needs to be a qualified physician supervising the hormone replacement therapy, and who can perform follow-up blood retests to monitor the progress of the treatment. Adrenal Fatigue in a Nutshell; People suffering adrenal fatigue, are tested many times for levels of cortical/cortisol and are found to have very low-normal levels and even clinically low levels. They do however, pass the ACTH Stimulation test, the one most often used to detect severe adrenal diseases and this test rules out true adrenal insufficiency. To believe a patient needs no treatment because it is not full blown adrenal hypofunction, is in my opinion a disservice to these patients, who suffer very real symptoms from this adrenal fatigue syndrome. What treatments help patients with adrenal fatigue? The more basic treatments are those the patient can do with some effort involving their own lifestyle. Getting more rest and sleep can be tremendously helpful, cutting back and even eliminating stimulants from the diet, such as too much sugar, caffeine, alcohol and tobacco, can also help greatly. Reducing stress, through relaxation and pursuit of enjoyable activities that allow for stress reduction, can help as well. Exercising to your tolerance level, can also help build up the adrenals and the body in general but exercise must not be overdone but increased gradually at a safe and helpful pace. Supplements that can also be very helpful, in building up adrenal function, include good multivitamins, the "B" vitamins (especially B-12), vitamin C, magnesium and zinc. You can also take short-term over-the-counter supplements to add to your vitamins, such as DHEA - which is another adrenal hormone that will convert into other needed hormones (including the sex ones), adrenal glandular - which is animal based adrenal extract containing adrenal gland tissue and licorice root extract, which helps the body produce higher levels of cortical. I would strongly caution however, that you take such supplements as recommended by the manufacturers of them, following all their warnings and directions. I experienced adrenal fatigue as previously mentioned and it became, more severe when I also experienced the onset of autoimmune thyroid disease (Hashimoto's) that caused me hypothyroidism.

My adrenal fatigue over time and together with the thyroid disease caused me to also experience Chronic Fatigue Syndrome. Even with thyroid medication treatment, I have had to work on my adrenals. Repeated tests I had done to check my adrenal hormone levels, revealed very low cortical levels for over a year period. In fact, some of these readings were clinically low. I did however pass an ACTH Stimulation test, ruling out adrenal insufficiency. Even Medical Doctors looking at these test results, admitted that my cortical was very low but they would also tell me there was no treatment available for sub-clinically low adrenal gland function. I began using the treatments I listed earlier in this article and I began to see significant improvement, which I maintain to this day (as shown in my blood cortical levels). I now only take a good multi-vitamin, having weaned off the other adrenal supplements, plus I do take medication for hypothyroidism. I do resort to the adrenal supplements when the support is needed - when chronic fatigue and/or that stressed-out feeling returns. I still must be cautious because overwork, too much stress and inadequate rest/sleep, can result in setbacks for me. I don't experience them as severely or nearly as often, as I did before I understood the cause and before implementing the lifestyle practices and treatments. I also believe my needing to take more care in this area, is due to the thyroid disease, which I also take treatment for - "Amour Thyroid" Natural hormone replacement medication. If you feel you may be suffering from adrenal fatigue, talk to your Doctor about it. You might even consider seeing a Holistic MD, a Naturopath physician or an Osteopath Doctor, as these types of physicians, more often recognize this very real syndrome.

SIX

Mean Spirited Ignorant People Place Stigmas on The Disabled

I will be commenting in this article on a note a young lady placed on Facebook in regard to people who pre-judge (scoff) at others who have need to use a government issued handicap sign for use of handicap disabled parking spaces. Her note goes along with other stigmas directed at the severely physically challenged. I therefore used her truly wise article to type one of my own on similar subject-matter (as a disabled person).   Now, to the subject-matter. - - -

{This first paragraph is a general commentary on the hatefulness that has developed in the human population. Afterward, below this, I go into the "handicap stigmas", this article is titled regarding.} GENERAL COMMENTARY: Most of the US population and most likely people in other countries as well are witnessing the attitudes of people having changed dramatically over the past few decades. This is especially true of the last decade to date and I have even heard radio show hosts talk about it on many occasions. Jesus Christ himself stated that in the last days (at the part of mankind's current dispensation, that *"And because iniquity shall abound, the love of many shall wax cold."* (Matthew 24:12).

Christ in his wisdom, was giving us a picture in this end-times sermon, demonstrating the past love mankind had for each other as being like a candle that has soft or liquefied wax on/in it that hardens after being burned. With each passing year, that wax becomes more hardened and hardened hearts are incapable of genuine love. The cure of course is to become *"a new creature in Christ"* (2 Corinthians 5:17) or to renew their fellowship with Christ Jesus and allow him to *"shed abroad his love in their hearts through the Holy Spirit"* (Romans 5:5).

I have a handicap hang-sign for my front mirror; however, I only use it if there's not parking already close enough to get in and out of the place I'm going into. I have Stage 2 non-smoker related COPD, a ruptured disc about mid-spine and an inch-long cyst in my lower spine (near tailbone), stage 4 deteriorated knee cartilage and shoulder rotator cuff deterioration, Mitral Valve Prolapse in my heart, among a few other things, I have days of symptom flares and some days of feeling relatively normal. On bad days I'm grateful for my handicap parking "privilege". I've had the exact same thing happen with "the looks" - some even have a half-way laugh type smile on their face. If they could feel one of our worse days just once, I don't believe they would display their "righteous indignation" ever again.

The Government doesn't give these signs out without solid proof of one's disabilities, so these people shouldn't call the Government stupid when they deem a person "disabled/Handicapped". For many of us, we mask our symptoms when possible, therefore people often remark "he doesn't look sick to me". I'll also mention that the wanna-be he-men types make statements like (excuse the bluntness but this is a true example). *"By God I sure wouldn't get a government hand-out, I would keep working even if I had to crawl to get it done"* …*pilgrim*. Ignorance can sure run deep in some people. *"The lips of the righteous feed many: but fools die for want of wisdom."* (Proverbs 10:21).

SEVEN

Death from Medical Errors a Huge Growing Problem

In a video produced by my wife and I, we talk about the very serious problem of deadly medical errors. We have given our extremely important message with anonymity for everyone with exception of ourselves. It is true regardless of this fact. Many people within our own relatively small circle of friends, have had negative medical experiences and all reputable medical information websites state that medical errors are the 3rd leading cause of death in America. This an is alarming statistic and some of the medical groups studying the causes of medical errors, which includes a major consideration called "doctor burn out", also state that the overall problem is getting worse.
--
While we should have empathy for doctors that are overworked, overbooked and burnt-out, we cannot slight the damaging and sometimes fatal results of it. Patients who have become ill and are simply wanting doctors who have the compassion to want to see them well. This, rather than being sloughed-off, ridiculed, resented and in worse health conditions than they had before seeing doctors of the type just described. There certainly are good doctors and great doctors out there but patients must be proactive in observing any signs that a doctor is a burned out one. This is where "second opinions" come in and simply "switching doctors", both of which happen every day in our country. So, a patient must be proactive in making sure their doctor is hearing their concerns and questions. The National Institutes of Health ran a radio commercial not long ago and that may still be aired today. It states that "Patients should express their needs in detail to their health providers because in their

words "If the patient is not communicating their needs, their doctor will clam-up."

--

Some doctors actually despise hearing patients make suggestions because they don't have their level of intelligence. Others, however, want to hear everything a patient desires to express but when doctor visits have a goal of being timed at 8-Minutes (true of some doctor's offices), this is a goal much harder to achieve. Patients must be proactive as stated previously but if they believe in prayer, they should also engage in it and ask God to remove any hindrances or confusion. Even with these things being done, they must always be willing to search for better doctors and second opinions on diagnoses.

EIGHT

Results of My Ethnicity Test through Ancestry DNA

(This was the first DNA testing I've had done, followed by two others which I cover in other articles to come. Did you know that *"the hobby of people seeking their genetics, is the 2nd most popular following gardening?"* - Spencer Wells: Bachelor of Science in Biology, University of Texas and PhD in Biology, Harvard.)

I did ethnicity testing through the ancestry.com company, plus two more I will also post articles about, that show me having less British/Irish and more of the other ethnicities listed in this first article. Ancestry.com has a U.S. testing lab that is purported to be near 100% accurate in determining ethnicities, using many 100s of 1,000s of DNA markers. The program is headed by PhD scientists specializing in genomics and bioinformatics. People provide vials of saliva mixed with a stabilizing/preserving solution and they then send the sample to the DNA testing lab. The testing analysis is for maternal and paternal ethnicity via "Autosomal DNA". Formerly, testing labs offered only Y-chromosome or Mitochondrial DNA testing which only gave maternal or paternal analysis, but labs have developed new methods for testing both. The tests result for me shows I'm of 47% Great Britain ethnicity and 27% Ireland. NOTE: I will be getting re-tested through a different DNA lab, toward the end of September 2015. This first test left me a 4th (26%) of my ethnicity from elsewhere, which they determined the origins of on my remaining test results, that I will list following.

I was disappointed that my rumored Native American DNA was simply not there on this test. I believe the test results I will obtain in late September 2015 may show otherwise and if so, I will explain why I believe a new test will show a small percent of American Indian. I have an MD cousin - a historian who tediously and systematically traced my "Lowrance" surname ancestry, to the family of "Saint Lawrence of Rome" ("Lawrence" being the Latin version of Lowrance). Our ancestors were of either Italy, France or Spain (likely a mix). The name "Lowrance", literally means "Man of Laurentius" - a city on the west coast of the Italian Peninsula southwest of Rome, "the original capital of the Latins" according to Wikipedia. It turns out that other parts of my slightly more ancient DNA ethnicity, does indeed include Italy, France and Spain These are areas the ancestry DNA testing people circled analytically, on European maps - one of which showed Italy centrally, another showing Spain centrally and a third showing France centrally. France, Spain and Italy are also encompassed/included on the analytical maps of 'Great Britain', 'Italy', 'The Iberian Peninsula' and 'Europe West'. With these inclusions, this raises Spain (mapped 3 times), France (Mapped 4 times) and Italy (mapped 5 times) as origins of my ancestry, to a higher level.

So, am I part Spaniard, French or Italian? ...Probably all three but most of my DNA is British and Irish, with Scandinavian and Finn (Finland) being included (NOTE: My 3rd test shows only 45% British/Irish, which will be posed in a future article). There is a small amount of Asian mixed in as well - 2%. My Reaction to the Analytical Ethnicity Maps The 2% Asian DNA, with the analytical map showing India centrally and a large area of West China was a surprise! My highest percent ethnicity is Great Britain as mentioned previously, which didn't surprise me. France and part of Italy are also within the circle of the Great Britain analytical map, while these same countries are highlighted-centrally on others, which I found interesting and exciting. This was true of other maps as well, some of which also included Spain (highlighted centrally on one of the ethnicity maps). I called the ancestry DNA testing people and they said even lighter-highlighted, circled areas represent actual DNA ethnicity. So, even Great Britain adds more French and Italian into the mix, being within the circled areas of my DNA. These countries are on the other mapped DNA areas as well (e.g. 'Europe West' and 'Iberian Peninsula'), the latter two mentioned, also showing 'Spain' and 'Italy' again.

I felt that the combination of these facts showed very interesting ancestry in my background. Some people might say "but no one has that many ethnicities", however, some of these ethnic groups likely go back 100s or even 1,000s of years in my family tree. My very small amount of Asian Indian DNA (2%) could have easily been a British soldier ancestor who married an Asian woman. There was rapid expansion of British power through the greater part of the Indian subcontinent in the early 19th century. The Italian, European-Spanish, French, Scandinavian and Finland also likely go further back in my ancestry than does my UK and Irish DNA. Regardless, I still have some of the DNA from those ancestors, who over time. Migrated to different countries, intermarrying with these different ethnic groups. They eventually settled in Britain and Ireland for a long period of time and then on to the United States. I am a Caucasian-American (a typical white guy) although some of my ancestors were somewhat darker-skinned people (e.g. Italian/Greek, Spaniard and Asian-Indian).

NINE

My Original Reason for Doing Three DNA Ancestral Tests

I was far less interested in finding very distant relatives with the 3 DNA tests I took; more than 20 generations away in my family history, or in branched-off cousins with fractions of a percent of DNA in common with mine. In my case I had a story within my ancestral history, per two family tree books written by my *PhD Medical Doctor* - Cousin, who searched-out this information within the most reputable archive-records libraries in the nation of the USA. I wanted to see if the ethnicities and ancestral countries involved in this world-changing story, were genuinely true.

Let me confess that I'm lazy because I tested only for ethnic backgrounds I have, with no follow-up on family tree development. I do have 2 family books written in the early 1960s by a doctor-cousin (plus 2 co-researchers), who traveled to the top records libraries in the U.S... However, these go back regarding my family ancestry, only about as far as the 16th century (with exception of our "Lowrance - surname origin" - 3rd century). That's similar in timeframe to what the DNA companies do.

The results I found from DNA testing, were confirmed as definitively as could possibly be, regarding the major ancestral story (e.g. surname origin and ancestral "French Huguenots"). I'm proud to have been able to do this confirmation by comparing 3 different ancestry tests I had done, to my family tree/history books that were began, starting with extensive research in 1960 (the book's print dates came slightly later in the 1960s). Of course, there were other surprises apart from this main story I was seeking to confirm, such as all 3 DNA tests showing me to have Asian ancestry, which likely points to Native American ancestry (according to new scientific genetics studies). Geneticists are involved in the Asian – Native American connection, with research being done currently. I will cover much more regarding my DNA ancestry in future articles.

I wrote a book after only 2 of the 3 DNA tests because I really had not decided to do a 3rd one. I did a 3rd test however so the book was a bit premature. I now have enough information to write a second short book (about eight to ten thousand words - similar in length to this one), which will discuss my DNA analysis which I have now had done through *4 companies* that analyze human Genomes! I've seen lots of videos and articles written by people saying the same type things regarding their Ancestry results not agreeing with their well-established family trees and ethnicities. This was the case with me as well, but I completed two other tests in addition to the "Ancestry" company's test. I also did the "23andme" and "Geographic 2.0 Next Generation" tests; the latter having the most impressive team of scientists and universities behind/conducting the DNA testing. What I was able to do was to compare all three and I did find very definite, unmistakable common threads. My crossover comparisons showed the Southern and Southern parts of Europe such as France, Italy, Germany, Iberian (Spain Portugal) and Scandinavia. All 3 also showed me to have 2.0% Asian, each probably being Native American. Their own information states this regarding Asian people emigrating to North America at an ancient time; mostly to the USA. Scientists are giving this lots of attention, this being the year 2017.

Most of these first major world countries I named above including France, were the Countries of "The Huguenots" (my ancestors) and their trek across Southern Europe, into Germanic countries,

Scandinavia, to Wales England and finally for many, into the USA. These "Protestant Reformation" people fled from extreme persecution, while spreading protestant doctrine. My direct well-established ancestors: named in my family tree books compiled in the early 1960s, are named in the list researched by *The National Huguenot Society.* "Johannes Lorentz" and family are one of them - Late 1700s to early 1800s, listed by NHS, as being "Qualified Huguenot Ancestors". He and his children are also named in our family tree books published approximately 50 years ago. Several of his children were the first to take-on my family's present and permanent surname - "Lowrance". In this sense the tests were very valuable to me, in gaining this confirming information but I feel time periods (various times of settlement and emigration) have much to do with the varied test results of these ancestral DNA companies. Example: The Nat. Geno 2.0 test shows me to be 45% British/Irish, while the Ancestry Company's test shows me to be 75%. The Ancestry Co. is likely showing one snapshot time while Nat Geno 2.0 is averaging several snapshot time periods in comparing my Genome to that of a vast number of other people.

For example, they may only be going back with a pool of DNA/Genome matches based on your Genome, from only 1 to 2 hundred years ago, this is going to show a lot of British/Irish. These countries were the last stops for so many European people before America branched-off and gained independence. If they go further back however, many people find they have Southern Europe, Eastern Europe, non-European countries, etc..., in their ancestral ethnicities. *SO*, my main point to this article regarding ancestral DNA testing companies, is that their analyses differ in many cases, due to how far back they go (100 to 500 years ago or even much more). So, my advice is to cross-compare a couple or 3, or even more tests to get a better ancestral picture (try to include one that shows your "Haplogroups"). I realize this means the cost of your ancestry search will be somewhat more significant, but the question is: "How important is it for you to know *the most possible* about your ancestral ethnicities that you can reasonably achieve?"

NOTE: I am not affiliated with any of these companies, in any way. I'm sure some people would disagree with my advice regarding being tested by more than one company. However, this is my honest opinion as to why they vary differently but likely significantly accurate at the same time, within the snapshot time-periods each look at. National Geographic's 2.0 Next Generation shows the most ancestral-ethnicity snapshots in my opinion and with the greatest scientific ancestry analysis. It did take me a while to understand that the different company's genome pools they've collected (each have close to a million of them) - they compare these with yours/ours, which differ in the number of people they have collected samples from for different countries. They may look for somewhat more recent ancestry-ethnicities or for somewhat more ancient analysis comparisons.

TEN

Does Hypothyroid Therapy Always Relieve Emotional Symptoms?

If you are hypothyroid (underactive thyroid), which causes a slowed/low metabolism and your symptom of depression is not lifting with hormone replacement therapy, I'm sorry to hear of your symptom struggles. I do want to encourage you that you are far from alone and I am included in the significant percent of treated hypothyroid patients with this problem. There are millions of thyroid patients with symptom struggles despite being on treatment and emotional symptoms of anxiety and depression are some of the most common. Doctors who are less updated on thyroid disease research will tell their patients that depression happens with hypothyroidism and anxiety with hyperthyroidism as if it's that's a simple, cut-and-dried fact that doesn't vary among patients. The fact is however that disordered anxiety is likely as common in hypothyroid patients as depression is, and for most patients it's a combination of the two. The autoimmune type hypothyroidism (Hashimoto's disease) also being the most common, can cause symptoms apart from normal hormone levels but treatment that is adequate or optimal with thyroid hormone replacement, can go a long way toward symptom relief and for some patients it gives them total relief of symptoms. I personally experienced relief in many areas within a few months of beginning on my own hypothyroid treatment - the emotional symptoms being the major ones. I still struggle with other symptoms due to co-morbid problems caused by my thyroid disease (i.e. musculoskeletal pain). Beginning a few years ago, the emotional symptoms raised their ugly heads again as well (Fluctuations in autoantibodies? – Possibly.). The symptom-relief that I have experienced has been greatly appreciated and a tremendous help to me for functioning better at work etc... NOTE: I began receiving S.S. Disability in 2012 when additional health disorders arose, including "non-smokers COPD" (yes it exits and 1,000s of people die from it yearly). A new dose takes eight weeks to adjust within the body, but this varies and also depends on dose changes you might also need. Doctors usually start at lower doses and titrate upward, increasing the dose slowly. They are tweaking the dose toward adequate/optimal levels, so you may be in for a dose increase or two before you see the better results. Once at the right level for you (determined by repeat blood retests), it can still take months to see it really do its job in your body, but you should see ongoing improvement as you go along. Doctors also don't always tell patients they may have some adjustment symptoms to the dose or side effects of their bodies adjusting to the hormone coming in from the outside (I wasn't). Your own thyroid slows its own production of hormones even more because of the hormone supplementation and you may reach a break-even point before improvement takes place. Many patients I've corresponded with - myself included in this fact, attest to having a worsening of their symptoms before they started improving.

It's a strange phenomenon but absolutely dose take place regardless of whether some doctors are aware of it or not. Patients fail to communicate which can otherwise help them recover a better quality of life. Patients who need the additional help of emotional stabilizing drugs or counseling/therapy, should not feel ashamed or embarrassed about it. *"And I will pray the Father, and he shall give you another Comforter, that he may abide with you forever"* (John 14:16 KJV - Quoted from Jesus referring to *spiritual* comfort).

ELEVEN

Being Refused Doctor Treatment for Illegitimate Illegal Reasons

Readers of this article will need to read my immediately preceding one titled: *"My Horrific Experiences with Certain Medicare Doctors"*. The reason being that this one is directly related to the other. Each will give better understanding to the other.

This one is a response I made to a doctor who, on the same day of only my second appointment with him, dismissed me as a patient by written letter. According to HIPAA and possibly COBRA laws, doctors are never supposed to refuse an established patient unless for highly legitimate reasons. This doctor's reason was due to my refuting his suggestion that there was nothing wrong with my lungs, when 5 years of consecutive testing shows very clearly that there is something to worry about, including symptoms. Hypochondria is attempting to be implied as the problem but when you read what my Pulmonary Function Tests (PFTs) are saying in the main body of this article below, this is a slough-off diagnosis (he supposedly reviewed all of these tests). It is one that spares a doctor in question, further investigation for "cause". Please read-on to understand what I mean by this. *{Note: I have had doctors diagnose COPD and sometimes Restrictive Lung Disease - the latter being the correct one but finding "cause" can mean the difference between me living longer or dying younger.}*

My Reply After Dismissal by the Doctor:
{The Letter} - - -
Dear Doctor,

You were anxious to send out the dismissal letter dated April 12th, 2017 (very same day as my 2nd office visit with you), with my next 'appointment' not being until December 2017. Your very first sentence (my wife being present) was "I don't think you have anything to worry about." The letter you sent to dismiss me, reveals to me that you are offended at patient feedback, especially if it is stated passionately. Yes, I did get somewhat forward with you after your remark saying "there's nothing really wrong" but you must understand I have been given this same runaround regarding my lung illness for *5 years*. Let a legally appointed doctor see my tests and see what answer you get from them. No one, but no one among Medicare MDs knows what it is. However, upon my calling The National Jewish Hospital and speaking to an NP on the phone twice, she said it was a rapid decline according to my ongoing PFT testing.

Her other advice to me was that a pulmonologist needed to find out what "the cause" was, instead of my being told "you have very minimal obstruction" (with 20 points drop in FEV1 and FVC separately and worsening symptoms). I've been told this minimal obstruction brush-off at each visit with doctors like you; board certified as pulmonologists. I've had at least 6 points drop in my FEV1 and FVC at every 6-month office visit and little to no response for it with bronchodilator use in an office test setting.

While I realize you don't like patients seeking knowledge online, my sources are always the top in the world – The National Institutes of Health, Medline Plus, Mayo Clinic, National Jewish Hospital, Medscape, Medicine.net, Merk Manual and WebMD. These sites have articles stating that restrictive lung disease presents exactly as mine does. The FVC/FEV1 ratio will be normal or even above normal but separately they're low. I have gone to 3 different Doctors (I have statements showing this), who I asked if I could get bronchoscopy but all three backed out, not having the time. My regular Dr. knows about these. He also knows that I went to a cardiologist who would not perform echocardiogram (a follow up one after 3 years - the previous showing several problems), and, *even with my appointment being set up for it* which was confirmed a second time before the appointment. The reason? Again, it was due to time constraints in my strongly held opinion. He didn't even listen to my heart with a stethoscope, just as you didn't listen to my lungs with yours on my 2nd visit (several months apart from the 1st visit with you) – my wife was with me for both.

The true problem? Doctors want smooth visits with patients and even though the NIH has a radio spot stating "Talk to the Dr. you're seeing, or they will clam up" (exact words). The AARP magazine I receive says "Do not accept 'it's just aging' or other sluff-off snap diagnoses, when you know you have something that needs further attention". This leads me to my decisive point. The NIH and other reputable sources state that the "Doctor Burnout" problem is severely bad. If you do a search on the subject, you'll see there are endless pages on this. One problem is that some doctors entered their profession with true intentions of abiding by their oath and because they literally do have compassion (like my Primary Care Physician). Others entered the profession simply as a career move. ...Which of these are you? Have you come to resent patients? Last of all, I have too many ailments/diseases (tests confirm this), that cause me daily suffering, to let the scariest one be sluffed-off – *"When you can't breathe, nothing else matters"* (American Lung Association).

My wife and I (married 34 years as of 2017), have family like everyone else, including 2 grown kids – the oldest, age 32, my

son who has given me a granddaughter (now age 11) and my age-27 daughter who is a coordinator at an office in OKC for people with substance abuse and domestic abuse problems. She has a master's but plans to get her Doctorate and PhD. This type information of a human life should wake up any doctor but if burnout is severe enough they will even detest this. Your very first words to us at the 2*nd and last* visit (again, my wife was there) were "I don't think you have anything to worry about". Therefore, I knew that very moment that you would not be my legitimate 2*nd* opinion pulmonologist. There is no need to transfer any records; your office never generated any and I have copies of all my past pulmonary records.
Cordially James Lowrance

Subheading (*Post Scriptum*)
This part of the article, covers spiritual aspects regarding doctors who lose their compassion for patients, which I believe to be brought about at least to some degree by the enemy of mankind, Satan's kingdom of hindering spirits:

Due to my having a lung disease problem, that has been called "asthma" by some Medicare doctors, "COPD" by others, possible "Pulmonary Hypertension" by some and "Restrictive Lung Disease" by yet others, it left me for years, wanting to know the true source of the problem. Everything has a cause and effect but these doctors who all had my very clear 'Pulmonary Functions Tests' to look at, showing 20 points drop in my most important lung functions, within a 4 to 5-year period. Example: FEV1 - a major test, went from being in the mid 80 points in year 2012 to a 20-point drop in the mid 60 points by year 2016. Symptoms-only are what was me to a pulmonologist in 2012 but my test ranges were normal back then. The same is true of the FVC - a 20-point drop in four years. The ratio of these two of course is normal (something doctors also highly-consider) because they are both at the same dwindling number, causing a normal ratio. {NOTE: *All doctors are not bad; many are excellent*, so if you're a medical professional please remember my stating this as you read the remainder of this article.}

It's like saying how do I get to 65% using two numbers? Well, you take 65 plus 65 which equals 130. You then divide that number by 2 and it equals 65 - that's *100% of the number* you wanted to arrive at. I had a doctor who only a few days ago, tell me that even with my main lung function numbers being mid 60% on FEV1 and FVC (varies from 65 to 67 depending on the PFT lab used), that because the ratio of the 2 together is normal, *all is well*. This is not true because a normal ratio between the two does not take away from the fact that the FEV1 and FVC, each separately, have dropped to a level that normally would represent "COPD stage 2". With the ratio between the two being normal, this does in fact rule out COPD but at the same time is highly indicative of **restrictive lung disease** (some forms are deadly within 5 years of diagnosis). One PFT I had done at a doctor's office had a computer-generated report/analysis, which stated "Restrictive Disease - Lung age 85", which of course concerned me but my doctor at this office (different city we lived in when my daughter was in college) was great. I liked him very much and he said, "Those analysis-readouts are not set in stone, so don't lose any sleep over it." However, like any normal person, I have suffered anxiety and depression ever since, but I cope with it quite well with God's help.

In fact there is a computer-generated graph of my flow volume loop that shows an abnormal flattening also indicating a restrictive lungs pattern. I have an upper right lobe nodule with stable scarring around it but my lungs (plural) have either

Atelectasis in them (areas of collapsed lung) or *Scarring*. I do have what I was told were minor heart problems, that could contribute to my breathing problem but has this possible connection been investigated? No, it has not...not even with my going to a pulmonologist, who sloughed me off and would not perform the test that I literally set the appointment for and confirmed with them by phone, before the office visit that I needed that specific test. I was supposed to get the test and there was no misunderstanding regarding my need for it but it still was not performed.

Because of these type battles with doctors, which should never occur, I have become a bit testy with *some* of them. Never with my PCP (regular Doctor) because he embodies what a true doctor should be, and he is, I will guess, about 60 years of age. In my opinion, if a doctor has not burned out by his 40s, he is not a 'career man only' but one who cares about people and the oath taken by him is also 'his calling'. The dilemma we also have in our USA nation, is a doctor shortage. This doubles-down on the difficulty in getting proper medical care because overbooked, continually rushed doctors are more apt to become one of the burnout statistics. The WebMD online site states *"Half (50%) of family doctors across all age categories said they had burnout in the 2015 report, up from 43% in 2013"*. If one looks at 2017 statistics, they are almost certainly higher than these numbers.

I have decided simply to live the best I can and let doctors slough me off whenever they like. When something gets bad enough, they'll simply put me in ICU, and I will die at a time of God's choosing. I have opted out of artificial life support and even resuscitation if it is obvious that being brought back to life means more suffering for me. This may sound morbid to some readers, however, the battles with doctors over the years has done as much damage to my health as anything else. I'm a burn out statistic from the other side of the coin; as a patient. When you have constant pain and other symptoms, including not being able to breath properly, you simply don't have the strength to battle doctor burn out. I will of course keep doing what my regular PCP asks me to do for the sake of my health. However, I will not battle specialists any longer, in attempt to get them to do the right thing. I ask God that he take them into his hands for the good or bad they do and I'll just continue to live on. That's really the best thing I can do after all that has transpired in the past. There's nothing better than God fighting my battles; He's far better at it than I am.

I will be posting a letter following this article, as a separate entry, that will be self-explanatory (I hope). It is in regard to my most recent but last battle with a specialist and/or a regular MD (I've also had to change PCPs for same reasons in the past). So, look for that posting that will likely appear above this article, since it will be a newer one. It is basically my response to this doctor writing a letter to me saying he no longer wanted me as a patient. Did I do something outrageous to make him slough me off completely? No, my wife was with me at both of my visits with him, she said I was straightforward at times but never raised my voice and certainly never threatened him. It was because I, as a patient suggested that certain things should be investigated.

He felt that by my doing this, I was disrespecting him as a doctor. I did also relate to him a negative experience I had with a cardiologist, so that he would suggest a different one. He said he already had planned to refer me to a colleague of his who is a cardiologist, but this will now never happen. As I said before it is in God's hands now, so I will simply let Him handle it from here. I will only do those simpler things, that I know are my duty to do (e.g. take meds my PCP prescribes and live as healthy as possible). Again, look for my next article - my letter of reply to a doctor who sloughed me off in writing. It contains some interesting information that most patients are unaware of but that they should be!

TWELVE

My Publications on Thyroid Myopathy and Neuropathy

I have written to a fair extent about how thyroid disease can affect nerve and muscle function. In one of the smaller books I took 6 detailed Q&A and made the booklet from them. "Thyroid Neuropathy and Myopathy Questions and Answers" is the title of that resource. I took the 6 questions from among those I have received through correspondence from thyroid patients, over the past decade or so (Since about 2004). I then compiled them into the booklet with relatively detailed answers. The questions that were asked of me were mostly those I received by email, from members of fellow patient support forums and message boards where I was moderator. They obtained my private email address of that time, by request. While I am not a medical professional, these fellow patients knew I was well-studied as a layperson but that most importantly "I had been there".

I had been and was in some of the same situations they were corresponding with me about. When some of these forums were discontinued and taken offline (not by hosting companies but by the owners of the websites), I gleaned some of my better forum responses on the thyroid-related myopathy and neuropathy subjects from them as well as from email correspondence previously-described. These are represented under the 'Q and A' headings within the booklet. Among the subjects of discussion that took place between me and these other thyroid patients, were symptoms of thyroid myopathy and/or neuropathy (the former being muscle weakness and the latter being nerve damage causing a variety of symptoms including pain). I am well-informed about the types of testing that were administered to me personally when I was being diagnosed with both myopathy and peripheral neuropathy. I have gained knowledge regarding these thyroid-related issues and the prognoses that can usually be expected from treatments for them (how patients respond to the treatments).

Within the discussions, I talk about blood tests and sometimes overlooked deficiencies of nutrients that can cause neuropathies and myopathies, which thyroid disease patients (and diabetics) are more susceptible to. I also look at both hypothyroid (underactive) and hyperthyroid (overactive) conditions, both of which can contribute to these symptom-problems of muscle weakness and nerve pain. Special types of testing involved in diagnosing these problems are also a point of discussion, including the QSART test, EMG and nerve/muscle biopsy testing. These discussions are for fellow-patient support and general educational purposes and thyroid patients should always follow their doctor's orders.

Being armed with some degree of knowledge in these areas, however, can help patients better discuss with their doctors, their options for controlling symptoms. Some patients may even overcome these manifestations of muscle weakness and nerve pain completely over time. This depends on correctable comorbid illnesses; additional hormone imbalances and/or vitamin deficiencies being treated. In some cases, physical therapy can restore muscle function considerably in some patients.

{Word Count 10,432}

END NOTE

Very few doctors have time to thoroughly educate their patients. The reputable information that is available online, usually requires searching multiple sites to find all the abridged, full-spectrum, layperson information needed by uninformed patients. When you are seriously ill, lengthy online search is not always the preferred option. Hopefully that statement will help those readers out there, complaining of layperson authors like me, covering medical information in books and articles. Especially with medical errors being the 3rd leading cause of death in the USA. I certainly hope it does quell their tone of disagreement because many of us who write these patient-to-patient booklets and books, have spent many years gleaning the best possible information to share with fellow patients. Mary Shomon for example, is the Nation's #1 Thyroid Disease Advocate and she has no medical credentials. She has however, written several New York Times Best Sellers on thyroid disease.
I too am a Patient Advocate.

James M. Lowrance